BE A VEGETARIAN

THE NATURAL WAY TO

A HEALTHY EVER YOUNG LIFE

Grayson O'Connell

Table of contents

Chapter I:

Introduction

Welcome to the world of vegetarianism, a lifestyle that embraces the power of plant-based eating for the betterment of your health and the planet. In this introductory chapter, we will explore the rise of vegetarianism, its impact on personal well-being, and the environment. Prepare to embark on a journey of discovery, as we delve into the purpose of this Book and the comprehensive guidance it offers for adopting a vegetarian lifestyle.

1.1 The Rise of Vegetarianism:

In recent years, there has been a remarkable surge in the popularity of vegetarianism. People from all walks of life are recognizing the benefits of embracing a plant-powered diet. We will explore the driving factors behind this rise, such as concerns for personal health, animal welfare, and environmental sustainability. Understanding the significant shift towards vegetarianism will lay the foundation for your own journey towards a compassionate and sustainable lifestyle.

1.2 Purpose of the eBook:

The purpose of this eBook is to provide you with a comprehensive resource to support your transition to a vegetarian lifestyle. We understand that embarking on this journey may seem daunting at first, but fear not! Our goal is to empower and guide you every step of the way. You will gain knowledge, practical tips, and delicious recipes to ensure a smooth and successful transition to vegetarianism.

1.3 Personal Health and the Environment:

Vegetarianism offers a multitude of benefits, both for your personal health and the environment. We will explore the scientific research that highlights the positive impacts of plant-based eating on reducing the risk of chronic diseases, improving overall well-being, and promoting longevity. Additionally, we will delve into the environmental consequences of animal agriculture and how adopting a vegetarian lifestyle can contribute to mitigating climate change, reducing water usage, and preserving natural resources.

1.4 What to Expect:

As you progress through this Book, you will gain a deeper understanding of the different types of vegetarian diets, including lacto-vegetarian, ovo-vegetarian, and vegan, and their respective variations. We will address common concerns and misconceptions about vegetarianism, offering reassurance and dispelling myths. You will find practical guidance on transitioning from a meat-based diet to a vegetarian one, including tips for stocking your pantry and kitchen essentials.

1.5 Navigating the Chapters:

This eBook is structured to provide you with a comprehensive and cohesive guide to vegetarianism. Each chapter builds upon the previous one, offering valuable information and practical advice to ensure a successful and fulfilling vegetarian journey. From understanding nutrition and meal planning to discovering delicious vegetarian recipes and addressing common challenges, every aspect of adopting a vegetarian lifestyle will be explored in depth.

Conclusion:

By embracing vegetarianism, you are making a positive impact on your own health and the world around you. This journey will open doors to new flavors, culinary adventures, and a greater connection with nature. Get ready to embark on this transformative path as we delve deeper into the world of vegetarianism, equipping you with the knowledge and inspiration to lead a vibrant, compassionate, and sustainable life.

Chapter 2:

Understanding Vegetarianism

In this chapter, we will delve into the concept of vegetarianism and gain a comprehensive understanding of its various forms and philosophies. By exploring the different types of vegetarian diets and the reasons why individuals choose this lifestyle, you will be equipped with the knowledge needed to make informed decisions about your own dietary choices.

2.1 Definition and Types of Vegetarian Diets:

To fully grasp the essence of vegetarianism, we will begin by defining what it means to be a vegetarian. We will explore the different types of vegetarian diets, such as lacto-vegetarian (including dairy products in the diet), ovo-vegetarian (including eggs in the diet), and vegan (excluding all animal products). Understanding the distinctions between these diets will enable you to identify which approach aligns best with your personal values and dietary preferences.

2.2 Ethical and Environmental Considerations:

Vegetarianism is often driven by ethical and environmental considerations. We will delve into the ethical aspects of vegetarianism, including the compassionate treatment of animals, the reduction of animal suffering, and the promotion of animal welfare. Additionally, we will explore the environmental impact of animal agriculture, such as deforestation, water pollution, and greenhouse gas emissions. By examining these considerations, you will gain insight into the broader implications of choosing a vegetarian lifestyle.

2.3 Health Benefits of Vegetarianism:

Vegetarianism has been associated with a wide array of health benefits. We will explore the scientific research that supports these claims, including the reduced risk of heart disease, hypertension, type 2 diabetes, obesity, and certain types of cancer. Furthermore, we will discuss the potential advantages of vegetarian diets in terms of weight management, improved digestion, and enhanced nutrient intake. Understanding the positive impact of vegetarianism on personal health will strengthen your motivation to adopt this lifestyle.

2.4 Meeting Nutritional Needs:

One concern often raised about vegetarian diets is whether they provide adequate nutrition. In this section, we will address common questions regarding nutrient deficiencies and share insights on how to meet your nutritional needs as a vegetarian. We will discuss key nutrients, such as protein, iron, calcium, omega-3 fatty acids, and vitamins, and explore plant-based sources that can fulfill these requirements. By understanding the principles of balanced nutrition in a vegetarian diet, you can ensure optimal health and well-being.

2.5 Transitioning to a Vegetarian Lifestyle: Transitioning from a meat-based diet to a vegetarian lifestyle can be a gradual process. In this section, we will provide practical guidance and strategies to facilitate a smooth transition. We will explore methods such as Meatless Mondays, flexitarianism, and incremental shifts, allowing you to find an approach that suits your personal preferences and circumstances. Additionally, we will offer tips on managing cravings, finding suitable alternatives, and dealing with potential social challenges that may arise during the transition period.

Conclusion:

Understanding the different types of vegetarian diets, their ethical and environmental considerations, and the associated health benefits provides a solid foundation for embracing a vegetarian lifestyle. By recognizing the diverse motivations behind vegetarianism and acquiring knowledge about meeting nutritional needs, you are empowered to make informed choices and embark on a fulfilling journey of compassionate and sustainable eating. In the next chapter, we will delve deeper into the practical aspects of transitioning to a vegetarian diet and setting up your kitchen for success.

Chapter 3:

Getting Started with Vegetarianism

Congratulations on your decision to embrace a vegetarian lifestyle! In this chapter, we will guide you through the initial steps of transitioning to a vegetarian diet. We will help you assess your motivations, address common concerns, and provide practical tips to ensure a successful and sustainable start to your vegetarian journey.

3.1 Assessing Your Motivations:

Understanding your motivations for adopting a vegetarian lifestyle is essential for long-term success. In this section, we will explore the various reasons individuals choose vegetarianism, such as health, environmental concerns, animal welfare, or personal beliefs. By reflecting on your own motivations, you will develop a strong foundation that will keep you motivated and committed to your new way of eating.

3.2 Addressing Common Concerns:

Embarking on a vegetarian journey may raise common concerns and questions. We will address these concerns and provide reassuring information to alleviate any doubts you may have. Topics such as protein intake, nutrient deficiencies, and meal variety will be explored, empowering you with the knowledge needed to confidently navigate your new vegetarian lifestyle.

3.3 Transitioning to a Vegetarian Diet:

Transitioning from a meat-based diet to a vegetarian diet is a gradual process that can be tailored to your individual needs and preferences. In this section, we will provide practical guidance on how to make the transition as smooth as possible. We will discuss strategies such as gradually reducing meat consumption, experimenting with vegetarian alternatives, and seeking support from vegetarian communities. With these tips, you can make a successful shift towards a plant-powered way of eating.

Some Advantages of a Vegetarian Diet

A vegetarian diet offers numerous advantages, ranging from personal health benefits to positive environmental and ethical impacts. Here are some key advantages of following a vegetarian diet:

Improved Heart Health: Vegetarian diets tend to be lower in saturated fats and cholesterol, which are commonly found in animal products. By focusing on plant-based foods rich in fiber, vitamins, and minerals, vegetarians have a reduced risk of heart disease, high blood pressure, and stroke.

Weight Management: Vegetarian diets, when properly balanced, can be effective for weight management and weight loss. Plant-based foods tend to be lower in calories and higher in fiber, which aids in maintaining a healthy weight.

Lower Risk of Chronic Diseases: Studies have shown that vegetarians have a reduced risk of developing chronic diseases such as type 2 diabetes, certain types of cancer (including colon, breast, and prostate cancer), and metabolic syndrome. The abundance of antioxidants and phytochemicals in plant-based foods may contribute to these protective effects.

Increased Intake of Nutrient-Rich Foods: Vegetarian diets often emphasize a wide variety of fruits, vegetables, whole grains, legumes, nuts, and seeds. These foods are rich in essential nutrients such as fiber, vitamins (including vitamin

C, vitamin E, and folate), minerals (such as potassium and magnesium), and antioxidants.

Environmental Sustainability: Animal agriculture is a significant contributor to greenhouse gas emissions, deforestation, and water pollution. By reducing or eliminating the consumption of animal products, vegetarians contribute to a more sustainable and environmentally friendly food system.

Ethical Considerations: Many people choose a vegetarian diet due to ethical concerns for animals. By opting for a plant-based diet, individuals can minimize their contribution to animal suffering and the exploitation of animals for food production.

Cultural and Culinary Exploration: Adopting a vegetarian lifestyle encourages individuals to explore a wide range of plant-based ingredients and cuisines from various cultures. This can expand culinary horizons, introduce new flavors, and foster creativity in the kitchen.

Economic Benefits: Vegetarian diets can be cost-effective, as plant-based proteins such as legumes, tofu, and tempeh tend to be more affordable compared to animal protein sources. Additionally, home-cooked vegetarian meals can be budget-friendly and reduce overall food expenses.

It's important to note that while there are numerous advantages to a vegetarian diet, it's essential to plan and ensure proper nutrient intake to meet individual nutritional needs. Consulting with a healthcare professional or registered dietitian can provide personalized guidance and support on adopting and maintaining a healthy vegetarian lifestyle.

3.4 Stocking Your Vegetarian Pantry:

A well-stocked vegetarian pantry is key to creating delicious and nutritious meals. We will guide you through the essentials of a vegetarian pantry, including grains, legumes, nuts, seeds, herbs, spices, and plant-based protein sources. You will learn how to create a versatile pantry that enables you to prepare a wide range of flavorful vegetarian dishes.

Having a well-stocked vegetarian pantry is just the first step. Knowing how to utilize the ingredients in your pantry effectively will help you create a wide range of delicious and nutritious vegetarian meals. Here are some tips on how to make the most out of your vegetarian pantry:

Plan Your Meals:

Take some time to plan your meals for the week or even just a few days in advance. This will help you determine which pantry items you need to use and allow you to create balanced and varied meals. Consider incorporating different grains, legumes, and vegetables to ensure a diverse and nutrient-rich diet.

Get Creative with Grains and Legumes:

Grains and legumes are versatile and can be the base for many vegetarian dishes. Experiment with different cooking methods and flavor combinations.

For example:

Cook quinoa or brown rice and use it as a base for Buddha bowls or stir-fries.

Make a hearty lentil stew or soup packed with vegetables and spices.

Try making homemade veggie burgers using a combination of beans, grains, and spices.

Use chickpeas or black beans to make flavorful vegetarian tacos or enchiladas.

Explore International Cuisines:

Your vegetarian pantry can help you explore various international cuisines. Here are some ideas:

Make a flavorful Indian curry using canned tomatoes, coconut milk, and spices like cumin, turmeric, and coriander.

Create a Mediterranean-inspired salad with canned chickpeas, olives, tomatoes, cucumbers, and a drizzle of olive oil and lemon juice.

Prepare a Thai stir-fry with tofu or tempeh, vegetables, and a sauce made from soy sauce, lime juice, and ginger.

Experiment with Herbs and Spices:

Herbs and spices can elevate the flavors of your vegetarian dishes. Don't be afraid to experiment and try new combinations. Some suggestions:

Add dried basil and oregano to tomato-based pasta sauces or sprinkle them on roasted vegetables.

Use cumin and paprika to season roasted chickpeas or add depth to Mexican-inspired dishes.

Incorporate turmeric and ginger into stir-fries, curries, or lentil dishes for a warm and earthy flavor.

Incorporate Nuts, Seeds, and Dried Fruits:

Nuts, seeds, and dried fruits can add texture, crunch, and sweetness to your vegetarian meals. Here are a few ideas:

Top your morning oatmeal or yogurt with a sprinkle of chopped nuts and dried fruits.

Add toasted sesame seeds or flaxseeds to salads, stir-fries, or homemade granola.

Make a homemade trail mix by combining different nuts, seeds, and dried fruits for a quick and nutritious snack.

Try Homemade Staples:

Take advantage of your pantry by making homemade staples like sauces, dressings, and spreads. For example:

Blend soaked cashews with nutritional yeast, lemon juice, and garlic to make a creamy vegan cheese sauce.

Make your own salad dressings using olive oil, vinegar, and herbs.

Create a homemade hummus using canned chickpeas, tahini, garlic, and lemon juice.

Experiment and Have Fun:

Don't be afraid to get creative in the kitchen and try new recipes. Use your pantry ingredients as a starting point and adapt recipes to your taste preferences. Modify recipes to include different vegetables, spices, or herbs based on what you have on hand.

Remember, your vegetarian pantry is a resource that allows you to create nourishing and delicious meals. Enjoy the process of cooking, exploring new flavors, and experimenting with different combinations. With a well-utilized pantry, you'll have endless possibilities to enjoy the variety and benefits of a vegetarian lifestyle.

3.5 Equipping Your Kitchen:

In addition to stocking your pantry, having the right kitchen tools and equipment will enhance your cooking experience as a vegetarian. We will explore essential kitchen tools, such as knives, cutting boards, cookware, and appliances, that will make meal preparation efficient and enjoyable. With a well-equipped kitchen, you'll be ready to embark on your culinary adventures as a vegetarian.

When adopting a vegetarian lifestyle, having a well-equipped kitchen can make all the difference in preparing delicious and nutritious meals.

Knives and Cutting Boards:

Invest in a set of high-quality knives that includes a chef's knife, a paring knife, and a serrated knife. These will be your go-to tools for chopping, slicing, and dicing vegetables, fruits, and herbs. Also, have a selection of cutting boards in different sizes to prevent cross-contamination when preparing various ingredients.

Cookware:

Having a few versatile and durable pieces of cookware will greatly enhance your cooking experience. Essential cookware items include:

Non-stick skillet or frying pan for sautéing vegetables and making stir-fries.

Saucepan and stockpot for boiling pasta, cooking grains, and preparing soups or stews.

Baking sheets or trays for roasting vegetables and baking.

Blender or Food Processor:

A blender or food processor is invaluable for preparing smoothies, sauces, dips, and dressings. It can also be used to grind nuts, make nut butter, or blend ingredients for soups and purees.

Mixing Bowls and Utensils:

A variety of mixing bowls in different sizes is essential for mixing ingredients, tossing salads, or marinating vegetables. Utensils such as spatulas, whisks, and wooden spoons are necessary for stirring, flipping, and mixing ingredients.

Baking Essentials:

If you enjoy baking, stock your kitchen with these baking essentials:

Measuring cups and spoons for precise measurements.

Mixing bowls for combining dry and wet ingredients.

Baking pans and sheets for cakes, cookies, and bread.

Rolling pin for flattening dough.

Wire cooling racks for cooling baked goods.

Slow Cooker or Instant Pot:

A slow cooker or Instant Pot can be a time-saving and convenient addition to your kitchen. These appliances allow you to effortlessly prepare soups, stews, and one-pot meals with minimal effort and time investment.

Vegetable Spiralizer:

A vegetable spiralizer is a handy tool for creating vegetable noodles or "zoodles" from zucchini, carrots, or other firm vegetables. It's a great way to incorporate more vegetables into your meals and create low-carb alternatives to pasta.

Grater and Zester:

A grater is useful for shredding cheese, grating vegetables like carrots or zucchini, and creating fine citrus zest for added flavor in dishes.

Storage Containers:

Invest in a variety of storage containers with tight-sealing lids to store leftovers, meal preps, and pantry staples. Glass containers are preferable for food safety and longevity.

Spice Rack:

A well-stocked spice rack is essential for adding flavor to your vegetarian dishes. Include commonly used spices like cumin, paprika, turmeric, chili powder, garlic powder, and dried herbs such as basil, oregano, and thyme.

Vegetable Peeler and Slicer:

A vegetable peeler is handy for peeling vegetables and fruits, while a mandoline slicer can create thin and uniform slices for salads or vegetable chips.

High-Speed Blender:

If you enjoy making smoothies, sauces, or creamy soups, consider investing in a high-speed blender.

It can effectively blend tough ingredients like nuts, seeds, and fibrous vegetables.

Remember, it's not necessary to have all these tools and equipment at once. Gradually build your kitchen arsenal based on your cooking preferences and budget. The goal is to have a functional kitchen that supports your vegetarian lifestyle and makes meal preparation a breeze.

Conclusion:

Getting started with vegetarianism involves understanding your motivations, addressing concerns, and making practical adjustments to your kitchen and pantry. By assessing your motivations and dispelling common concerns, you lay a solid foundation for your vegetarian journey. Stocking your pantry with essential ingredients and equipping your kitchen with the right tools will empower you to prepare delicious vegetarian meals with ease. In the next chapter, we will dive deeper into the world of vegetarian nutrition, ensuring that you receive the proper nutrients to support your health and well-being on your vegetarian path

Chapter 4:

Nutrition and Meal Planning

A well-planned vegetarian diet can provide all the necessary nutrients for optimal health. In this chapter, we will explore the importance of nutrition in a vegetarian lifestyle. We will discuss key nutrients, meal planning strategies, and tips for incorporating a variety of plant-based foods into your diet. By understanding the principles of vegetarian nutrition and mastering meal planning, you will be able to create balanced and satisfying meals that support your health and well-being.

4.1 Essential Nutrients in a Vegetarian Diet:

A balanced vegetarian diet should include a variety of nutrients to support your body's needs. We will delve into the essential nutrients commonly associated with vegetarian diets, such as protein, iron, calcium, omega-3 fatty acids, vitamin B12, and vitamin D. You will learn about plant-based sources of these nutrients and how to ensure you meet your daily requirements to maintain optimal health.

4.2 Protein in a Vegetarian Diet:

Protein is an essential component of any diet, and we will explore the various plant-based sources that can provide you with ample protein as a vegetarian. We will discuss complete protein sources, combining plant proteins to achieve complete amino acid profiles, and dispel the myth that vegetarians struggle to meet their protein needs. By understanding protein-rich plant-based foods, you can create satisfying and nourishing meals.

Protein is an essential nutrient that plays a crucial role in building and repairing tissues, supporting immune function, and maintaining overall health. Many people associate protein primarily with animal products, but it is entirely possible to meet your protein needs on a vegetarian diet. Here's how you can ensure an adequate protein intake:

Plant-Based Protein Sources:

Vegetarian diets offer a wide range of plant-based protein sources that can provide all the essential amino acids your body needs. Include the following protein-rich foods in your diet:

1: Legumes: Beans, lentils, chickpeas, and soy products like tofu, tempeh, and edamame are excellent   sources of protein.

2: Whole Grains: Quinoa, brown rice, oats, and whole wheat products like bread and pasta contribute to your protein intake.

3: Nuts and Seeds: Almonds, walnuts, cashews, chia seeds, hemp seeds, and flaxseeds contain protein and healthy fats.Dairy and Eggs (for lacto-ovo vegetarians): Milk, yogurt, cheese, and eggs are protein-rich options.

Combining Protein Sources:

While plant-based proteins can provide all the essential amino acids, it's beneficial to consume a variety of protein sources throughout the day. Combining different plant-based proteins can help ensure a more complete amino acid profile. For example:

Pairing legumes with whole grains: Combine beans or lentils with rice, quinoa, or whole wheat bread to create a complete protein source.

Mixing nuts or seeds with legumes: Sprinkle chopped almonds or sesame seeds on a lentil salad or add peanut butter to a chickpea curry.

Incorporating dairy or eggs (if applicable): Include dairy products like Greek yogurt, cottage cheese, or eggs in your meals for additional protein.

Pay Attention to Quantity:

It's important to consume an adequate amount of protein to meet your needs. The Recommended Daily Allowance (RDA) for protein is approximately 0.8 grams per kilogram of body weight for adults. However, individual protein requirements may vary depending on factors such as age, activity level, and overall health. Consulting with a registered dietitian can help determine your specific protein needs and guide you in achieving them.

Snack on Protein-Rich Foods:

Include protein-rich snacks in your daily routine to boost your protein intake. Some ideas include:

Greek yogurt with berries or a sprinkle of nuts.

Hummus or bean dip with veggie sticks.

Trail mix with nuts, seeds, and dried fruits.

Protein bars or energy balls made with plant-based protein powder.

Protein Supplements:

If you're finding it challenging to meet your protein needs through food alone, protein supplements can be an option. There are numerous plant-based protein powders available, such as pea protein, soy protein, and hemp protein. These can be added to smoothies, oatmeal, or used in recipes to boost protein content. However, it's always best to obtain nutrients from whole foods whenever possible.

Balancing Your Diet:

While protein is essential, it's important to maintain a well-balanced diet that includes a variety of other nutrients. Incorporate plenty of fruits, vegetables, whole grains, and healthy fats to ensure you're meeting your overall nutritional requirements.

Consult a Registered Dietitian:

If you have specific dietary concerns or are transitioning to a vegetarian diet, consulting a registered dietitian can provide personalized guidance. They can help you develop a meal plan that meets your nutritional needs and answer any questions or concerns you may have.

Remember, with proper planning and a diverse selection of plant-based protein sources, it is entirely possible to meet your protein needs on a vegetarian diet.

4.3 Iron and Calcium in a Vegetarian Diet:

Iron and calcium are important minerals that play vital roles in maintaining overall health. We will discuss plant-based sources of iron and calcium and explore ways to enhance their absorption. You will learn about the importance of vitamin C in iron absorption and the significance of combining calcium-rich foods with vitamin D for optimal calcium utilization. By incorporating these nutrients into your vegetarian diet, you can support bone health and ensure healthy blood production.

Iron and calcium are two vital minerals that play crucial roles in maintaining overall health. While they are commonly associated with animal-based foods, it is entirely possible to obtain these nutrients from plant-based sources in a vegetarian diet. Here's how you can ensure an adequate intake of iron and calcium:

Iron:

Iron is essential for the production of red blood cells and the transport of oxygen throughout the body. There are two types of dietary iron: heme iron, found in animal products, and non-heme iron, found in plant-based foods. Vegetarians can rely on non-heme iron sources to meet their iron needs. Here are some plant-based iron sources:

1. Legumes: Lentils, chickpeas, kidney beans, and soybeans are excellent sources of iron. Pair them with vitamin C-rich foods like citrus fruits or bell peppers to enhance iron absorption.
2. Leafy Greens: Spinach, kale, Swiss chard, and other dark leafy greens are rich in iron. Enjoy them in salads, stir-fries, or smoothies.
3. Whole Grains: Incorporate iron-rich grains such as quinoa, oats, fortified cereals, and whole wheat products into your meals.
4. Nuts and Seeds: Snack on iron-rich nuts like almonds, cashews, and pistachios. Include

seeds such as pumpkin seeds, sesame seeds, and flaxseeds in your diet.

5. Dried Fruits: Raisins, apricots, dates, and prunes are concentrated sources of iron. They make for healthy, portable snacks or can be added to cereals, baked goods, or trail mixes.

6. Iron-Fortified Foods: Check for iron-fortified plant-based products like breakfast cereals, bread, and plant-based meat alternatives. These can be additional sources of iron in your diet.

To enhance iron absorption, consider the following:

. Consume vitamin C-rich foods alongside iron-rich foods. For example, squeeze lemon juice over your leafy green salad or pair beans with a tomato-based sauce.

. Avoid consuming calcium-rich foods or supplements at the same time as iron-rich foods, as calcium can inhibit iron absorption. Instead, separate these sources by a few hours.

Calcium:

Calcium is crucial for maintaining strong bones and teeth, muscle function, and nerve transmission. While dairy products are commonly associated with calcium, vegetarians can obtain this mineral from various plant-based sources. Consider the following calcium-rich foods:

1. Leafy Greens: Incorporate calcium-rich greens such as kale, collard greens, bok choy, and broccoli into your meals.
2. Fortified Plant Milk: Opt for calcium-fortified plant milks like almond milk, soy milk, or oat milk. These can be used as a dairy milk alternative in recipes, cereals, or beverages.
3. Tofu and Tempeh: These soy-based products are often fortified with calcium. Include them in stir-fries, curries, or marinated and grilled dishes.
4. Seeds: Sesame seeds are particularly rich in calcium. Sprinkle them on salads, stir them into sauces, or use tahini (sesame seed paste) in dressings or spreads.
5. Nuts and Nut Butters: Almonds, Brazil nuts, and hazelnuts contain calcium. Enjoy them as snacks or use them in recipes.
6. Legumes: Some legumes, such as chickpeas and white beans, provide a moderate amount of calcium.

Remember the following tips for optimizing calcium absorption:

. Ensure an adequate intake of vitamin D, as it aids in calcium absorption. Exposure to sunlight and fortified plant-based products can help meet your vitamin D needs.

4.4 Omega-3 Fatty Acids in a Vegetarian Diet:

Omega-3 fatty acids are crucial for brain function and heart health. While fish is a common source of omega-3s, we will explore plant-based alternatives such as flaxseeds, chia seeds, walnuts, and algae-based supplements. You will learn about the different types of omega-3 fatty acids and how to incorporate them into your vegetarian meals to support your overall well-being.

Omega-3 fatty acids are a type of polyunsaturated fat that plays a crucial role in supporting heart health, brain function, and reducing inflammation in the body. While oily fish is a well-known source of omega-3s, vegetarians can still obtain these essential fats from plant-based sources. Here's how to incorporate omega-3 fatty acids into your vegetarian diet:

1.Chia Seeds:

Chia seeds are an excellent plant-based source of omega-3 fatty acids. They are also rich in fiber and antioxidants. Sprinkle chia seeds on top of cereals, yogurt, or salads, or use them in smoothies, baked goods, and puddings.

2.Flaxseeds and Flaxseed Oil:

Flaxseeds are another great source of omega-3s. Grind whole flaxseeds and add them to your meals or use flaxseed oil as a dressing for salads or drizzle it over cooked vegetables. Store flaxseed oil in the refrigerator to prevent it from going rancid.

3.Walnuts:

Walnuts are not only delicious but also contain a good amount of omega-3 fatty acids. Snack on a handful of walnuts, chop them up and sprinkle them on salads or cereals, or incorporate them into your baked goods for added crunch and nutty flavor.

4.Hemp Seeds and Hemp Oil:

Hemp seeds and hemp oil are rich sources of omega-3s, as well as protein and other essential nutrients. Sprinkle hemp seeds over your meals, blend them into smoothies, or use hemp oil as a finishing touch to your dishes.

5.Algal Oil Supplements:

Algal oil is derived from algae and is an excellent vegetarian alternative to fish oil. It provides a direct source of long-chain omega-3 fatty acids, such as DHA (docosahexaenoic acid) and EPA (eicosapentaenoic acid). Algal oil supplements are available in capsule form and can be a convenient way to ensure adequate omega-3 intake.

6.Seaweed:

Certain types of seaweed, such as nori, contain omega-3 fatty acids. Use nori sheets to wrap sushi or crumble them into salads, stir-fries, or soups for a boost of omega-3s and unique flavor.

7.Plant-Based Omega-3-Enriched Foods:

Some food products, such as plant-based milk, yogurt, and eggs, are fortified with omega-3 fatty acids. Check product labels to find options enriched with omega-3s.

Remember the following tips for maximizing omega-3 absorption and health benefits:

. Consume a balanced diet that includes a variety of plant-based omega-3 sources to ensure a diverse nutrient intake.

. Aim for a regular intake of omega-3-rich foods throughout the week rather than relying on one source alone.

. Store omega-3-rich foods properly to maintain their freshness and prevent rancidity.

. Discuss any dietary concerns or considerations with a healthcare professional or registered dietitian to ensure you are meeting your specific nutritional needs.

By incorporating these plant-based sources of omega-3 fatty acids into your vegetarian diet, you can enjoy the numerous health benefits associated with these essential healthy fats.

4.5 Creating Balanced Vegetarian Meal Plans:

Meal planning is an essential aspect of maintaining a healthy vegetarian lifestyle. We will discuss strategies for creating balanced meal plans that meet your nutritional needs. You will learn how to incorporate a variety of fruits, vegetables, whole grains, legumes, nuts, and seeds into your meals. We will also provide practical tips for meal prepping, batch cooking, and ensuring variety in your daily meals. With these meal planning techniques, you can enjoy a diverse and nutritionally balanced vegetarian diet.

Creating a balanced vegetarian meal plan is an essential part of ensuring that your body gets the nutrients it needs. With a little bit of planning, it's easy to create a vegetarian meal plan that's both delicious and nutritionally balanced.

Here are some tips on creating a balanced vegetarian meal plan:

1.Include a variety of vegetables: Vegetables are a great source of vitamins, minerals, and fiber. Include a variety of vegetables in your meals to ensure that you're getting a wide range of nutrients. Aim for at least 5 servings of vegetables per day.

2.Include plant-based proteins: Plant-based proteins, such as beans, lentils, tofu, and tempeh, are an important part of a vegetarian meal plan. These foods are high in protein, fiber, and other nutrients. Aim for at least 3 servings of plant-based proteins per day.

3.Include whole grains: Whole grains, such as brown rice, quinoa, and whole wheat bread, are an excellent source of fiber, B vitamins, and minerals. Aim for at least 3 servings of whole grains per day.

4.Incorporate healthy fats: Healthy fats, such as those found in nuts, seeds, avocados, and olive oil, are an important part of a balanced diet. Aim for 1-2 servings of healthy fats per day.

5. Pay attention to portion sizes: While vegetarian foods are generally healthy, it's important to pay attention to portion sizes to ensure that you're not overeating. Use a smaller plate and listen to your body's hunger and fullness cues.

6. Consider nutrient supplements: It's possible to get all the nutrients you need from a vegetarian diet, but some people may benefit from supplements. Speak to your healthcare provider to determine if you need to take any supplements.

Here's an example of a balanced vegetarian meal plan:

Breakfast: Whole grain toast with avocado and scrambled tofu, orange slices

Snack: Apple slices with almond butter

Lunch: Lentil soup with whole grain bread, mixed green salad with balsamic vinaigrette

Snack: Carrot sticks with hummus

Dinner: Black bean tacos with salsa, guacamole, and brown rice

Dessert: Fresh berries with whipped coconut cream

Remember, creating a balanced vegetarian meal plan is all about variety and balance. Experiment with different vegetables, plant-based proteins, and whole grains to create meals that are both nutritious and delicious.

4.6 Special Considerations: Athletes, Pregnant Women, and Children:

Vegetarianism can be adapted to meet the specific needs of different populations, including athletes, pregnant women, and children. We will discuss the unique nutritional considerations for these groups and provide guidance on meeting their dietary requirements while following a vegetarian lifestyle. Understanding these special considerations will empower you to cater to the needs of your body and those of your family members.

The vegetarian diet can offer a range of benefits for athletes, pregnant women, and children when planned carefully to ensure proper nutrient intake. Here are some benefits specific to each group:

1.Athletes:

Improved cardiovascular health: Plant-based diets tend to be lower in saturated fats and cholesterol, which can promote heart health and reduce the risk of cardiovascular diseases.

Enhanced recovery: Vegetarian diets can provide an abundance of antioxidants and anti-inflammatory compounds found in fruits, vegetables, and whole grains. These nutrients can help reduce exercise-induced inflammation and promote faster recovery.

Sufficient protein intake: Contrary to common misconceptions, it is possible for athletes to meet their protein needs through a well-planned vegetarian diet. Plant-based protein sources such as legumes, tofu, tempeh, and quinoa can provide the necessary amino acids for muscle repair and growth.

Increased fiber intake: Vegetarian diets are typically high in dietary fiber, which aids digestion, regulates blood sugar levels, and promotes satiety. This can help athletes maintain a healthy body weight and manage energy levels.

2. Pregnant Women:

Adequate nutrient intake: A well-planned vegetarian diet can provide pregnant women with all the necessary nutrients, including folate, iron, calcium, and vitamin D. These nutrients are vital for fetal development and maternal health.

Lower risk of gestational diabetes: Plant-based diets, especially those rich in whole grains, legumes, and vegetables, have been associated with a reduced risk of developing gestational diabetes during pregnancy.

Reduced exposure to contaminants: Some contaminants, such as mercury found in certain fish, can be harmful to the developing fetus. By avoiding animal products, pregnant women can minimize their exposure to these potential contaminants.

3. Children:

Balanced nutrition: A properly planned vegetarian diet can provide children with all the essential nutrients needed for growth and development. It can promote a diverse intake of fruits, vegetables, whole grains, and plant-based proteins, ensuring a wide range of vitamins, minerals, and fiber.

Establishing healthy eating habits: Introducing children to a vegetarian diet early in life can help them develop a taste for a variety of plant-based foods and establish healthy eating habits that may carry into adulthood.

Lower risk of obesity and chronic diseases: Vegetarian diets that focus on whole, unprocessed foods can help children maintain a healthy weight and reduce the risk of obesity-related conditions such as type 2 diabetes and cardiovascular diseases.

Regardless of the life stage, it's important to approach a vegetarian diet with careful planning to ensure sufficient intake of key nutrients. Consulting with a healthcare professional or registered dietitian can help tailor the vegetarian meal plan to meet specific nutritional needs and ensure a healthy and balanced diet.

Conclusion:

Nutrition is a critical aspect of a successful vegetarian lifestyle. By understanding the essential nutrients in a vegetarian diet, incorporating protein-rich plant-based foods, and ensuring adequate intake of iron, calcium, and omega-3 fatty acids, you can maintain optimal health. Furthermore, by creating balanced vegetarian meal plans and considering special dietary needs, you can customize your diet to support your individual requirements. In the next chapter, we will take a delicious turn and explore a collection of vegetarian recipes that will inspire and satisfy your taste buds.

Chapter 5:

Delicious Vegetarian Recipes

In this chapter, we will dive into the world of vegetarian cuisine and explore a collection of mouthwatering recipes. Whether you're a seasoned cook or new to the kitchen, these recipes will inspire you to create delicious, satisfying, and nourishing meals. From breakfast delights to satisfying main courses and delectable desserts, we have a variety of recipes that will tantalize your taste buds and showcase the diverse flavors and textures of vegetarian cooking.

5.1 Breakfast and Brunch Recipes:

Start your day off right with a selection of vegetarian breakfast and brunch recipes. From savory options like tofu scramble, vegetable frittatas, and avocado toast to sweet treats such as blueberry pancakes, overnight oats, and fruit smoothie bowls, these recipes will energize you and set the tone for a fantastic day ahead.

Tofu scramble

Tofu scramble is a popular vegan alternative to scrambled eggs that offers several health benefits. Here are some advantages of including tofu scramble in your diet:

1.Plant-based protein: Tofu is made from soybeans and is an excellent source of plant-based protein. It provides all the essential amino acids necessary for proper muscle growth, repair, and overall health. Tofu scramble can be a great option for individuals following a vegetarian or vegan diet or those looking to reduce their consumption of animal products.

2.Nutrient-rich: Tofu is a good source of various essential nutrients. It contains iron, calcium, magnesium, and B vitamins like vitamin B6 and folate. These nutrients are important for maintaining healthy blood cells, supporting bone health, and facilitating various metabolic processes in the body.

3.Heart-healthy: Tofu is low in saturated fat and cholesterol, making it a heart-healthy food choice. Consuming tofu as part of a balanced diet may help reduce the risk of heart disease and improve overall cardiovascular health.

4.Lower in calories: Tofu scramble is generally lower in calories compared to traditional scrambled eggs. This can be beneficial for individuals aiming to manage their calorie intake, support weight loss, or maintain a healthy body weight.

5.Versatility: Tofu scramble is highly versatile and can be customized to suit various flavor preferences. It can be seasoned with a variety of herbs, spices, and vegetables, allowing for a wide range of taste profiles. This versatility makes tofu scramble a versatile option for breakfast, brunch, or even as a filling for sandwiches or wraps.

6.Cholesterol-free: As tofu is derived from plants, it is naturally free of cholesterol. Consuming tofu scramble instead of scrambled eggs can be particularly beneficial for individuals with high cholesterol levels or those aiming to reduce their cholesterol intake.

When preparing tofu scramble, consider using organic, non-GMO tofu and incorporating plenty of vegetables for added nutrients and flavor. Experimenting with different seasonings and spices can also help create a flavorful and satisfying dish.

Blueberry pancakes

Blueberry pancakes can be a delicious and nutritious addition to your breakfast or brunch. Here are some benefits of enjoying blueberry pancakes:

1.Nutrient-rich: Blueberries are packed with vitamins, minerals, and antioxidants. They are a great source of vitamin C, vitamin K, and manganese. Antioxidants in blueberries, such as anthocyanins, help protect the body against oxidative stress and inflammation.

2.Fiber content: Blueberries are high in dietary fiber, which promotes healthy digestion and helps maintain regular bowel movements. Including blueberries in pancakes adds fiber to your meal, contributing to a feeling of fullness and supporting digestive health.

3.Brain health: Blueberries have been associated with Improved brain health and cognitive function. The antioxidants and phytochemicals in blueberries may help protect the brain from oxidative stress and reduce the risk of age-related cognitive decline.

4.Heart health: Blueberries are known to be heart-healthy due to their high content of antioxidants and flavonoids. Regular consumption of blueberries has been linked to a reduced risk of heart disease, as they may help lower blood pressure, improve cholesterol levels, and support healthy blood vessel function.

5.Mood-boosting properties: Blueberries contain compounds that may positively impact mood and mental well-being. Studies have suggested that consuming blueberries may help reduce symptoms of depression and anxiety and improve overall mood.

6.Versatile and delicious: Blueberry pancakes are not only nutritious but also a delightful treat. The burst of sweetness from the blueberries complements the fluffy texture of the pancakes, making them a satisfying and enjoyable breakfast option.

It's worth noting that the overall nutritional value of blueberry pancakes can vary depending on the recipe and additional ingredients used. To maximize the health benefits, consider using whole grain flour or incorporating other nutritious ingredients like Greek yogurt or flaxseeds into the pancake batter. And while blueberry pancakes can be a nutritious choice, moderation and balance in your overall diet remain important for optimal health.

5.2 Appetizers and Snacks:

Whether you're hosting a gathering or simply looking for a tasty snack, these vegetarian appetizer recipes will impress your guests and satisfy your cravings. Explore dishes like crispy vegetable spring rolls, homemade hummus with fresh veggies and pita chips, stuffed mushrooms, and flavorful guacamole with tortilla chips. These appetizers will keep your taste buds entertained and your hunger at bay.

Appetizers and snacks are an enjoyable part of any meal or gathering. They can offer a burst of flavor, provide a quick energy boost, and keep hunger at bay. Here's a closer look at appetizers and snacks, including their benefits and some ideas for delicious options:

Benefits of Appetizers and Snacks:

1.Satisfying hunger: Appetizers and snacks can help curb hunger between meals, providing a quick and convenient way to satiate cravings and maintain energy levels.

2. Socializing and entertaining: Appetizers are often served before a meal as a way to welcome guests and set the mood for a gathering. They encourage mingling, conversation, and a relaxed atmosphere.

3. Portion control: Snacks and appetizers can be portioned out to help manage overall calorie intake. By offering smaller portions, they allow for variety without overindulging.

4. Nutrient boost: Well-planned appetizers and snacks can contribute to a well-rounded diet by

providing an opportunity to include additional fruits, vegetables, whole grains, lean proteins, and healthy fats.

5. Culinary exploration: Appetizers and snacks provide an opportunity to explore different flavors, ingredients, and cuisines. They can introduce new tastes and textures, broadening culinary horizons.

Ideas for Appetizers and Snacks:

1.Fresh vegetable platter with dip: Offer a colorful assortment of raw vegetables like carrot sticks, cucumber slices, bell pepper strips, and cherry tomatoes. Pair them with a healthy dip like hummus, guacamole, or Greek yogurt-based tzatziki.

2.Bruschetta: Top slices of toasted baguette or whole-grain bread with a mixture of diced tomatoes, fresh basil, garlic, olive oil, and balsamic vinegar. It's a classic Italian appetizer bursting with flavor.

3.Stuffed mushrooms: Fill mushroom caps with a mixture of breadcrumbs, herbs, garlic, and cheese (or vegan alternatives), and bake until golden and crispy. They make delicious bite-sized appetizers.

4.Mini falafel: Prepare bite-sized falafel balls made from chickpeas and herbs. Serve them with a tangy tahini sauce or wrap them in pita bread with fresh vegetables for a wholesome snack.

5.Fruit skewers: Thread a variety of fresh fruits like strawberries, melon chunks, grapes, and pineapple onto skewers for a colorful and refreshing appetizer or snack. They are great for summer gatherings.

6.Baked tortilla chips with salsa: Make your own crispy tortilla chips by baking corn tortillas until lightly golden. Serve them with homemade salsa, which can be made from diced tomatoes, onions, jalapeños, cilantro, lime juice, and spices.

Remember to consider dietary restrictions or preferences of your guests when planning appetizers and snacks. It's always a good idea to offer a mix of options, including vegetarian, vegan, gluten-free, or nut-free choices, to accommodate various dietary needs and preferences.

5.3 Flavorful Main Courses:

Prepare to be amazed by the array of flavorful vegetarian main course recipes. From hearty vegetable stews and comforting pasta dishes to creative plant-based burgers and vibrant stir-fries, these recipes will prove that vegetarian meals can be both filling and satisfying. Indulge in dishes like chickpea curry, spinach and feta stuffed shells, lentil shepherd's pie, and tofu stir-fry with colorful vegetables.

5.4 Wholesome Salads:

Salads need not be boring, and these recipes will showcase the beauty and versatility of vegetarian salads. Discover vibrant combinations of fresh greens, colorful vegetables, protein-rich legumes, and delicious dressings. Try salads like quinoa and roasted vegetable salad, Greek salad with tofu feta, black bean and corn salad, and roasted beet and goat cheese salad. These wholesome salads will leave you feeling nourished and satisfied.

5.5 Satisfying Soups:

Warm up with a bowl of hearty vegetarian soup. These recipes will introduce you to a world of flavors and textures. Delight in creations like creamy tomato basil soup, lentil and vegetable soup, butternut squash and apple soup, and spicy coconut curry soup. These soups are not only comforting but also packed with nutrition, making them a perfect choice for a satisfying meal.

Satisfying soups are a comforting and nourishing addition to any meal. They can be enjoyed as a starter or even as a complete meal on their own. Here's a closer look at the benefits of satisfying soups and some ideas for creating delicious and fulfilling options:

Benefits of Satisfying Soups:

1.Hydration: Soups are typically broth-based, which means they have a high-water content. Consuming soups can contribute to your daily hydration needs and help maintain proper fluid balance in the body.

2.Nutrient-rich: Soups often contain a variety of vegetables, legumes, whole grains, and lean proteins, making them a great source of essential nutrients like vitamins, minerals, fiber, and antioxidants. They can help meet your daily nutrient requirements and support overall health.

3.Satiety and portion control: The high water and fiber content in soups can help create a feeling of fullness and satiety. Enjoying a bowl of soup before a meal or as a meal itself can help control portion sizes and prevent overeating.

4.Digestive health: Soups, especially those made with vegetables and legumes, are rich in dietary fiber. Fiber promotes healthy digestion, aids in regular bowel movements, and supports a healthy gut microbiome.

5.Warm and comforting: Soups provide a sense of warmth and comfort, especially during colder months or when you need a soothing meal. They can help you relax and unwind while enjoying a delicious and nutritious bowl of goodness.

Ideas for Satisfying Soups:

1.Vegetable Minestrone: A hearty and satisfying soup loaded with a variety of vegetables, beans, and whole-grain pasta. It's flavorful, packed with nutrients, and can be customized with your favorite veggies and herbs.

2.Lentil Soup: Lentils are a great source of plant-based protein and fiber. Combine them with aromatic vegetables, such as onions, carrots, and celery, and simmer them with vegetable broth and spices for a satisfying and nutritious soup.

3.Creamy Tomato Basil Soup: A classic favorite that combines the tanginess of tomatoes with the freshness of basil. Use ripe tomatoes or canned tomatoes, blend them until smooth, and add a touch of cream or coconut milk for a creamy texture.

4.Moroccan Chickpea Stew: A fragrant and hearty stew featuring chickpeas, warming spices like cumin and coriander, and vegetables like sweet potatoes, carrots, and tomatoes. It's a filling and flavorful option with a hint of exotic flavors.

5.Thai Coconut Curry Soup: This soup combines the creaminess of coconut milk with the vibrant flavors of Thai curry paste. Add vegetables, tofu, or your choice of protein for a satisfying and aromatic soup with a spicy kick.

6.Mushroom Barley Soup: A rich and earthy soup made with tender mushrooms, hearty barley, and aromatic herbs. It's a comforting option that can be enjoyed as a full meal or as a starter to a larger dinner.

Remember to adjust the seasoning and ingredients to suit your taste preferences and dietary needs. Soups can be versatile, so feel free to experiment with different vegetables, spices, and protein sources to create your own satisfying and nourishing creations.

5.6 Delectable Desserts:

No meal is complete without a sweet ending, and these vegetarian dessert recipes will leave you craving more. Indulge in treats like chocolate avocado mousse, fruit crumbles, banana bread, and vegan chocolate chip cookies. These desserts are not only delicious but also demonstrate the versatility of vegetarian ingredients in creating delectable sweet treats.

Delectable desserts are a delightful way to end a meal or indulge in a sweet treat. Whether you're a fan of rich chocolate, fruity flavors, creamy textures, or baked delights, there is a dessert to satisfy every craving. Here's a closer look at the benefits of delectable desserts and some ideas to make your taste buds dance:

Benefits of Delectable Desserts:

1.Enjoyment and indulgence: Desserts provide a moment of pure enjoyment and allow you to indulge your sweet tooth. Treating yourself to a delicious dessert can be a mood booster and a source of happiness.

2.Variety of flavors and textures: Desserts come in a wide range of flavors, textures, and presentations, allowing you to explore different tastes and experiences. From creamy and smooth to crunchy and gooey, desserts offer a variety of sensory pleasures.

3.Social bonding: Sharing desserts with loved ones can create a sense of togetherness and joy. Desserts often serve as a centerpiece for celebrations and gatherings, encouraging connection and camaraderie.

4.Creative expression: Dessert making is an opportunity for creativity in the kitchen. From decorating cakes to experimenting with flavor combinations, desserts allow you to showcase your culinary skills and express your unique style.

Ideas for Delectable Desserts:

1.Chocolate Mousse: A decadent and velvety dessert made from melted chocolate and whipped cream or aquafaba (chickpea brine for a vegan alternative). Serve it in elegant glasses and top with fresh berries or shaved chocolate for a luxurious touch.

2.Fresh Fruit Tart: A vibrant and refreshing dessert featuring a buttery crust filled with creamy custard and topped with an assortment of fresh fruits. It's a beautiful and light option that showcases the natural sweetness of fruits.

3.Classic Cheesecake: A rich and creamy dessert made with cream cheese, eggs, and a buttery graham cracker crust. Customize it with various toppings such as fruit compote, chocolate ganache, or caramel sauce for added decadence.

4.Warm Apple Crumble: A comforting dessert that combines baked apples with a crumbly topping of flour, oats, butter, and brown sugar. Serve it with a scoop of vanilla ice cream or a dollop of whipped cream for a delightful contrast of textures.

5.Tiramisu: An Italian favorite featuring layers of espresso-soaked ladyfingers, mascarpone cream, and a dusting of cocoa powder. It's an elegant and indulgent dessert that balances the flavors of coffee and creamy sweetness.

6.Homemade Ice Cream: Create your own flavors of ice cream using a base of cream, milk, sugar, and your choice of add-ins like chocolate chips, nuts, fruits, or cookie dough. Experiment with unique combinations to suit your taste preferences.

Remember to balance indulgence with moderation and consider personal dietary restrictions or preferences when enjoying desserts. Feel free to adapt recipes to accommodate dietary needs, such as using alternative sweeteners, gluten-free flours, or vegan substitutes. Whether you choose to make elaborate desserts from scratch or opt for quick and easy recipes, delectable desserts are sure to add a touch of sweetness and joy to your dining experience.

Conclusion:

Vegetarian cuisine is vibrant, flavorful, and diverse. This chapter has provided you with a range of delicious vegetarian recipes to explore. From breakfast to dinner and everything in between, these recipes will satisfy your taste buds and showcase the exciting possibilities of vegetarian cooking. Experiment with these recipes, adapt them to your preferences, and let your culinary creativity shine. Remember, vegetarianism is not only about what you're leaving behind but also about the incredible flavors and nourishment you can discover on your journey. In the next chapter, we will address common challenges and provide tips to help you stay motivated and overcome obstacles on your vegetarian path.

Chapter 6:

Overcoming Challenges and Staying Motivated

While embracing a vegetarian lifestyle can be rewarding, it is not without its challenges. In this chapter, we will address common obstacles that individuals may encounter on their vegetarian journey and provide strategies to overcome them. Additionally, we will explore tips to stay motivated, find support, and maintain a positive mindset to ensure long-term success in your vegetarian lifestyle.

6.1 Navigating Social Situations:

Eating vegetarian in social settings can sometimes be challenging, particularly when dining out or attending gatherings. We will discuss strategies for navigating these situations, such as researching vegetarian-friendly restaurants, communicating your dietary preferences with friends and family, and offering to bring a vegetarian dish to gatherings. By being proactive and assertive, you can ensure that your vegetarian choices are respected and accommodated in social settings.

Navigating social situations as a vegetarian can sometimes present unique challenges, but with a few strategies in mind, you can confidently navigate these scenarios while still enjoying social interactions. Here are some explained strategies to help you navigate social situations as a vegetarian:

1.Communicate your dietary preferences: Let your friends, family, and hosts know about your dietary choices ahead of time. Informing them in advance allows them to accommodate your needs and plan accordingly. Be clear and polite when explaining your vegetarianism and any specific restrictions or preferences you have.

2.Offer to contribute: If you're attending a gathering or event where food will be served, offer to bring a vegetarian dish or two. This ensures that there will be options available for you and others who may have dietary restrictions. It also shows your willingness to participate and contribute to the occasion.

3.Be prepared: If you're uncertain about the food options that will be available, consider eating something before the event to ensure you're not hungry. Additionally, carry some vegetarian-friendly snacks with you, such as nuts, granola bars, or dried fruits, in case there aren't many suitable options available.

4.Research restaurants and menus: Before dining out with friends or colleagues, research restaurants in advance and review their menus. Many establishments now offer vegetarian options or can accommodate dietary requests. Choosing a restaurant that caters to various dietary preferences ensures everyone can find something suitable to eat.

5.Be open to compromise: In certain situations, it may not be possible to find strictly vegetarian options. In these cases, be flexible and willing to make compromises based on your comfort level. You can focus on the side dishes, salads, or request adaptations to existing menu items to make them vegetarian-friendly.

6.Educate and share: Use social situations as an opportunity to educate others about vegetarianism, its benefits, and the variety of delicious vegetarian dishes available. If someone expresses interest or curiosity, be open to discussing your dietary choices and sharing your favorite vegetarian recipes or restaurants.

7.Practice assertiveness and respect: If someone offers you non-vegetarian food or questions your choices, respond assertively but respectfully. You can politely decline their offer and explain your reasons for being vegetarian without passing judgment on their choices. Remember, it's important to maintain a positive and understanding attitude in these situations.

8.Seek support and connect with like-minded individuals: Surround yourself with friends, family, or communities who understand and respect your vegetarian lifestyle. Connecting with like-minded individuals can provide support, recipe ideas, and a sense of belonging.

Remember, each social situation is unique, and it's essential to approach them with an open mind and positive attitude. By being proactive, communicative, and adaptable, you can navigate social gatherings while honoring your vegetarian values and enjoying the company of others.

6.2 Dealing with Cravings and Food Temptations:

Cravings for familiar non-vegetarian foods can arise during your transition to a vegetarian lifestyle. We will explore ways to deal with these cravings and temptations, such as finding suitable vegetarian alternatives, experimenting with new flavors and ingredients, and seeking support from fellow vegetarians. By exploring the rich variety of vegetarian cuisine, you can satisfy your cravings while staying committed to your dietary choices.

Dealing with cravings and food temptations is a common challenge when trying to maintain a balanced and healthy diet. Whether it's a sudden desire for something sweet, salty, or indulgent, understanding how to manage these cravings is key to staying on track with your goals. Here are some strategies to help you navigate cravings and food temptations:

1.Identify the trigger: Recognize what triggers your cravings. It could be stress, boredom, specific environments, or certain emotions. By understanding the underlying cause, you can find healthier alternatives to address those triggers rather than turning to food.

2.Practice mindful eating: Slow down and pay attention to your body's hunger and fullness cues. When a craving strikes, take a moment to pause and assess whether you're truly hungry or if it's a momentary desire. Mindful eating can help you differentiate between physical hunger and emotional cravings.

3.Plan and prepare: Plan your meals and snacks in advance to ensure you're adequately nourished throughout the day. Include a balance of macronutrients (carbohydrates, protein, and healthy fats) in your meals to keep you satisfied. Having healthy options readily available can help reduce impulsive and unhealthy choices when cravings arise.

4.Opt for healthier alternatives: Instead of completely denying yourself the foods you crave, seek healthier alternatives. For example, if you're craving something sweet, reach for a piece of fruit or a small portion of dark chocolate. If you're craving something crunchy and salty, try roasted chickpeas or air-popped popcorn.

5.Distract yourself: Engage in activities that divert your attention away from cravings. Go for a walk, read a book, listen to music, or call a friend. By occupying your mind and body, you can often overcome cravings without giving in to them.

6.Practice portion control: If you're truly craving a specific food, give yourself permission to indulge but practice portion control. Enjoy a small serving or a single serving of your desired food instead of completely depriving yourself. Savor the taste and eat it mindfully, allowing yourself to fully enjoy the experience.

7.Manage stress: Stress can often lead to emotional eating and intense cravings. Find healthy ways to manage stress such as exercise, meditation, deep breathing, or engaging in activities that bring you joy and relaxation. By reducing stress levels, you can better manage cravings triggered by emotional states.

8.Seek support: Reach out to friends, family, or a support group who can provide encouragement and understanding during moments of temptation. Having someone to talk to or share your experiences with can help you stay motivated and accountable.

Remember, occasional indulgences are a part of a balanced lifestyle. It's important to find a balance between satisfying your cravings and maintaining a nutritious diet. By adopting these strategies and developing a healthy relationship with food, you can better manage cravings and make mindful choices that align with your overall well-being.

6.3 Overcoming Nutritional Concerns:

Some individuals may have concerns about meeting their nutritional needs on a vegetarian diet. We will revisit key nutrients and discuss practical strategies to ensure a well-rounded and nutritionally balanced diet. You will learn about monitoring your intake of protein, iron, calcium, and other essential nutrients, and incorporating a variety of plant-based foods to meet your dietary requirements. By staying informed and making mindful food choices, you can address any nutritional concerns with confidence.

Being a vegetarian can provide numerous health benefits, but it's important to be mindful of potential nutritional concerns that may arise from eliminating certain animal products from your diet. By understanding these concerns and taking proactive steps to address them, you can ensure you're meeting your nutritional needs as a vegetarian. Here are some key nutritional concerns and strategies for overcoming them:

1.Protein intake: Protein is essential for tissue repair, muscle growth, and overall health. As a vegetarian, it's important to include plant-based sources of protein such as legumes (beans, lentils, chickpeas), tofu, tempeh, seitan, quinoa, nuts, seeds, and whole grains in your diet. Aim to include a variety of these protein-rich foods throughout the day to meet your protein needs.

2.Iron deficiency: Plant-based sources of iron, known as non-heme iron, are not as readily absorbed by the body compared to heme iron found in animal products. However, you can enhance iron absorption by consuming vitamin C-rich foods alongside iron-rich foods. Include citrus fruits, bell peppers, tomatoes, broccoli, and leafy greens in your meals. Additionally, consider cooking with cast-iron cookware, which can increase iron content in your meals.

3.Vitamin B12: Vitamin B12 is primarily found in animal-based foods, so it's important for vegetarians to ensure they're getting adequate amounts of this nutrient. Include fortified foods like plant-based milks, breakfast cereals, and nutritional yeast in your diet. Alternatively, you may need to consider a B12 supplement to meet your requirements. Consult with a healthcare professional for personalized guidance.

4.Omega-3 fatty acids: While fish is a common source of omega-3 fatty acids, vegetarians can obtain these essential fats from plant-based sources like flaxseeds, chia seeds, hemp seeds, walnuts, and algae-based supplements. Incorporate these sources into your diet to support brain health and reduce inflammation.

5.Calcium and vitamin D: Calcium is important for bone health, and vitamin D aids in calcium absorption. Include calcium-rich foods such as leafy greens, broccoli, fortified plant-based milk, tofu, and almonds in your diet. Additionally, ensure adequate vitamin D levels through exposure to sunlight or consider a vitamin D supplement if needed.

6.Zinc and iodine: Some vegetarian diets may be lower in zinc and iodine, which are important for immune function and thyroid health, respectively. Include foods like whole grains, legumes, nuts, seeds, and seaweed to increase your intake of these nutrients. Additionally, consider using iodized salt in moderation to meet your iodine needs.

7.Planning balanced meals: To overcome nutritional concerns, focus on creating well-rounded, balanced meals that incorporate a variety of whole plant-based foods. Include fruits, vegetables, whole grains, legumes, nuts, seeds, and plant-based proteins in your meals. Consider consulting a registered dietitian who specializes in vegetarian nutrition to help you create a personalized meal plan.

8.Stay informed and educated: Keep up with current research and information about vegetarian nutrition to ensure you have the latest knowledge. Stay connected with reputable resources, read books, and consult professionals to ensure you're making informed choices about your diet and nutrition.

Remember, everyone's nutritional needs may vary, so it's important to listen to your body and consult with a healthcare professional or registered dietitian for personalized advice and guidance. By being mindful of these nutritional concerns and implementing appropriate strategies, you can thrive on a vegetarian diet and enjoy optimal health and well-being.

6.4 Finding Support and Community:

Having a support system and connecting with like-minded individuals can greatly enhance your vegetarian journey. We will explore ways to find support and build a sense of community, such as joining vegetarian or vegan groups, participating in online forums or social media communities, attending vegetarian events or potlucks, and connecting with friends or family members who share similar dietary choices. By surrounding yourself with supportive individuals, you can share experiences, seek advice, and stay motivated in your vegetarian lifestyle.

6.5 Motivation and Mindset:

Maintaining motivation is crucial for long-term success as a vegetarian. We will discuss strategies to stay motivated and cultivate a positive mindset. Setting clear goals, reminding yourself of your reasons for choosing a vegetarian lifestyle, and celebrating milestones and achievements can help keep you motivated and committed. Additionally, practicing self-care, mindfulness, and gratitude can contribute to a positive mindset and overall well-being on your vegetarian path.

Transitioning to a vegetarian diet can be challenging, but it can also be a rewarding and fulfilling experience. Here are some strategies to help you stay motivated and cultivate a positive mindset as a vegetarian:

1.Clarify your reasons: Understanding your reasons for becoming a vegetarian can help you stay motivated and committed to your new lifestyle. Take some time to reflect on your values, goals, and health concerns, and write down why you've chosen to adopt a vegetarian diet. This can serve as a reminder when you encounter challenges or doubts.

2.Focus on the benefits: Instead of focusing on what you're giving up, focus on the benefits of your vegetarian lifestyle. This might include improved health, reduced environmental impact, and ethical considerations. Remind yourself of these benefits regularly, and celebrate your progress and achievements.

3.Connect with others: Seek out support from other vegetarians, whether it's through online communities, local meetups, or social events. Being part of a like-minded community can provide encouragement, inspiration, and practical advice. You can also share your experiences and challenges with others, and learn from their perspectives.

4.Experiment with new recipes and foods: One of the most exciting aspects of vegetarianism is the opportunity to explore new foods and flavors. Take advantage of this by trying new recipes, cuisines, and ingredients. You may discover new favorite foods and cooking techniques, and expand your culinary repertoire.

5.Plan ahead: Planning ahead can help you stay on track with your vegetarian diet, especially when faced with busy schedules or social events. Make a meal plan for the week, stock up on essential ingredients, and pack snacks and meals when you're on the go. Having a plan can reduce stress and help you make mindful choices.

6.Practice self-care: Taking care of your physical and mental health is essential for staying motivated and positive. Make time for regular exercise, sleep, and stress management techniques such as meditation or yoga. Prioritizing self-care can help you feel more energized, focused, and resilient.

7.Keep learning: Stay curious and open-minded about vegetarianism, and continue to learn about nutrition, ethics, and environmental issues. Read books and articles, watch documentaries, and attend events and workshops. This can help you stay informed, engaged, and motivated to make a positive impact.

Remember, cultivating a positive mindset and staying motivated as a vegetarian is a process that requires patience, flexibility, and self-compassion. Focus on progress, not perfection, and celebrate your successes along the way. With these strategies, you can enjoy the benefits of a vegetarian lifestyle while maintaining a positive and fulfilling outlook.

6.6 Embracing Flexibility and Progress:

Remember that adopting a vegetarian lifestyle is a journey, and it's okay to embrace flexibility and acknowledge progress along the way. We will explore the concept of flexitarianism, which allows occasional consumption of animal products, and discuss the importance of celebrating small victories and being kind to yourself throughout your vegetarian journey. By adopting a flexible and compassionate approach, you can navigate challenges, stay motivated, and continue to evolve in your vegetarian lifestyle.

Conclusion:

Overcoming challenges and staying motivated are essential for a successful and fulfilling vegetarian journey. By employing strategies to navigate social situations, manage cravings, address nutritional concerns, find support, and maintain a positive mindset, you can overcome obstacles and stay committed to your vegetarian lifestyle. Remember, the path to vegetarianism is unique for each individual, and embracing flexibility and progress is key. By staying motivated and open-minded, you can continue to experience the numerous benefits of a compassionate and sustainable way of eating. In the final chapter, we will reflect on your journey and provide tips for sustaining your vegetarian lifestyle for the long term

Chapter 7:

Frequently Asked Questions

As you embark on your vegetarian journey, it's natural to have questions and seek guidance along the way. In this chapter, we will address some of the most frequently asked questions about vegetarianism. From nutritional concerns to practical considerations, we will provide answers and insights to help you navigate your vegetarian lifestyle with confidence and clarity.

7.1 Is a vegetarian diet nutritionally balanced?

One common concern is whether a vegetarian diet can provide all the necessary nutrients. We will revisit the topic of vegetarian nutrition, emphasizing the importance of a well-planned diet that includes a variety of plant-based foods. By understanding key nutrients and implementing proper meal planning, you can ensure that your vegetarian diet is nutritionally balanced.

A vegetarian diet can be nutritionally balanced when it includes a variety of nutrient-dense plant-based foods that provide all the essential nutrients needed for good health. Here are some key nutrients to focus on when planning a nutritionally balanced vegetarian diet:

1.Protein: Protein is essential for building and repairing tissues in the body. Vegetarians can obtain protein from plant-based sources such as legumes, nuts, seeds, soy products, whole grains, and vegetables. Including a variety of these protein sources in your meals throughout the day can ensure you are meeting your daily protein needs.

2.Iron: Iron is important for the production of red blood cells and oxygen transport in the body. Plant-based sources of iron include legumes, leafy green vegetables, tofu, tempeh, nuts, seeds, and fortified cereals and grains. To enhance iron absorption, pair iron-rich foods with a source of vitamin C such as citrus fruits, bell peppers, or tomatoes.

3.Calcium: Calcium is essential for building strong bones and teeth. Vegetarians can obtain calcium from plant-based sources such as leafy greens, tofu, tempeh, fortified plant milks, and calcium-set tofu. Aim for three to four servings of calcium-rich foods daily to meet your calcium needs.

4.Vitamin B12: Vitamin B12 is important for nerve function and red blood cell formation. As vitamin B12 is primarily found in animal-based foods, vegetarians should include fortified plant milks, fortified cereals, and nutritional yeast to ensure adequate intake of this nutrient. Alternatively, consider taking a vitamin B12 supplement.

5.Omega-3 fatty acids: Omega-3 fatty acids are important for heart health and brain function. Vegetarians can obtain omega-3 fatty acids from plant-based sources such as chia seeds, flax seeds, hemp seeds, walnuts, and algae-based supplements.

6.Zinc: Zinc is important for immune function, wound healing, and DNA synthesis. Vegetarians can obtain zinc from plant-based sources such as legumes, nuts, seeds, whole grains, and fortified cereals.

To ensure a nutritionally balanced vegetarian diet, focus on incorporating a variety of whole, nutrient-dense plant-based foods throughout the day. Use online resources or consult with a registered dietitian to develop a personalized meal plan that meets your individual nutrient needs and preferences. With careful planning and attention to key nutrients, a vegetarian diet can provide all the essential nutrients needed for good health.

7.2 Where do vegetarians get their protein from?

Protein is a vital component of a healthy diet, and we will explore various plant-based sources of protein. From legumes and tofu to quinoa and nuts, you will discover a wide range of protein-rich options available to vegetarians. We will also discuss the concept of combining different plant proteins to ensure complete amino acid profiles.

7.3 What about iron and calcium in a vegetarian diet?

Iron and calcium are important minerals, and we will delve deeper into plant-based sources of these nutrients. You will learn how to incorporate iron-rich foods, such as leafy greens, beans, and fortified grains, into your meals. We will also explore calcium sources like tofu, fortified plant-based milk, and certain leafy greens to support bone health.

7.4 Can children and pregnant women follow a vegetarian diet?

We will address the suitability of a vegetarian diet for children and pregnant women. While vegetarianism can be appropriate for these groups, special considerations must be taken to ensure proper nutrient intake. We will provide guidance on meeting nutritional requirements and discuss the importance of consulting with healthcare professionals for personalized advice.

Yes, children and pregnant women can follow a vegetarian diet with careful planning to ensure they are meeting their nutrient needs. However, it is important to consult with a healthcare provider and a registered dietitian to ensure the diet is nutritionally adequate and appropriate for individual needs.

For children, a well-planned vegetarian diet can provide all the necessary nutrients for growth and development. However, it is important to ensure they are receiving adequate amounts of protein, iron, calcium, vitamin B12, and omega-3 fatty acids. Including a variety of plant-based protein sources such as legumes, nuts, seeds, soy products, and whole grains throughout the day can help meet protein needs. Iron-rich foods such as dark leafy greens, tofu, tempeh, and fortified cereals can help meet iron needs. Calcium-rich foods such as calcium-set tofu, leafy greens, and fortified plant milks can help meet calcium needs. Vitamin B12 can be obtained from fortified plant milks and cereals, or from a vitamin B12 supplement. Omega-3 fatty acids can be obtained from sources such as chia seeds, flax seeds, and algae-based supplements.

For pregnant women, a well-planned vegetarian diet can provide all the necessary nutrients for a healthy pregnancy. However, it is important to ensure they are receiving adequate amounts of protein, iron, calcium, vitamin B12, and folate. Including a variety of plant-based protein sources such as legumes, nuts, seeds, soy products, and whole grains throughout the day can help meet protein needs. Iron-rich foods such as dark leafy greens, tofu, tempeh, and fortified cereals can help meet iron needs. Calcium-rich foods such as calcium-set tofu, leafy greens, and fortified plant milks can help meet calcium needs. Vitamin B12 can be obtained from fortified plant milks and cereals, or from a vitamin B12 supplement. Folate is important for fetal development and can be obtained from sources such as leafy greens, legumes, and fortified cereals. Pregnant women may also need additional nutrients such as vitamin D and iodine, which can be obtained from fortified plant milks and iodized salt, respectively.

Overall, with careful planning and attention to nutrient needs, children and pregnant women can follow a vegetarian diet that is nutritionally adequate and supports good health. It is important to work with a healthcare provider and a registered dietitian to ensure individual needs are being met and to make any necessary adjustments to the diet.

7.5 What about omega-3 fatty acids on a vegetarian diet?

Omega-3 fatty acids are crucial for overall health, and we will explore vegetarian sources of these essential fats. From flaxseeds and chia seeds to algae-based supplements, you will discover alternative options to meet your omega-3 needs without relying on fish or fish oil.

7.6 How can I handle social situations as a vegetarian?

Navigating social situations can be a challenge, but we will provide strategies to help you handle them with ease. Tips for dining out, attending events, and communicating your dietary preferences will be discussed. You will also learn how to engage in constructive conversations and educate others about vegetarianism without judgment.

7.7 Can I still enjoy international cuisines as a vegetarian?

Absolutely! We will explore how to adapt international cuisines to suit a vegetarian diet. From Mediterranean dishes to Asian delicacies, you will discover ways to substitute meat with plant-based alternatives and enjoy the flavors of different cultures while staying true to your vegetarian lifestyle.

Absolutely! Being a vegetarian doesn't mean you have to miss out on enjoying international cuisines. In fact, many global culinary traditions offer a wide array of vegetarian dishes that are flavorful, diverse, and satisfying. With a little exploration and creativity, you can indulge in the rich flavors and unique dishes from around the world. Here are some tips to help you enjoy international cuisines as a vegetarian:

1.Research vegetarian-friendly options: Before dining out or traveling, take the time to research vegetarian-friendly restaurants or specific dishes within a particular cuisine. Many popular cuisines like Indian, Mediterranean, Thai, and Mexican have a wealth of vegetarian options available. Look for dishes that are traditionally vegetarian or can be easily modified to be vegetarian-friendly.

2.Explore plant-based protein sources: Different cuisines have their own plant-based protein sources that are central to their dishes. For example, Indian cuisine offers a wide range of vegetarian options with lentils, chickpeas, and paneer (a type of Indian cheese). Thai cuisine often features tofu and tempeh, while Mediterranean cuisine includes dishes with legumes like falafel and hummus. Embrace these unique ingredients and experiment with incorporating them into your meals.

3.Adapt recipes: Many international recipes can be modified to be vegetarian-friendly by substituting meat with plant-based alternatives or adding extra vegetables. For instance, you can swap meat for tofu or tempeh in stir-fries or curries, use vegetable broth instead of meat broth in soups, or substitute beans for meat in Mexican dishes like tacos or enchiladas. Don't be afraid to get creative and experiment with flavors and textures.

4.Communicate your dietary preferences: When dining out or attending social gatherings, communicate your dietary preferences clearly to chefs or hosts. They may be able to provide vegetarian options or suggest modifications to existing dishes. Additionally, informing your friends and family about your vegetarian lifestyle can help them accommodate your needs when planning meals or events.

5.Explore vegetarian-friendly food blogs and cookbooks: There are numerous vegetarian food blogs and cookbooks available that focus on international cuisines. These resources provide a wealth of recipes and inspiration for recreating authentic flavors at home. Experiment with different recipes and adapt them to suit your taste preferences.

6.Learn about vegetarian traditions: Some cultures have a long history of vegetarianism or have specific vegetarian dishes that are an integral part of their culinary heritage. Take the opportunity to learn about these traditions and explore their vegetarian offerings. For example, in Buddhism, vegetarianism is practiced by many, and Buddhist cuisine offers a variety of vegetarian dishes.

Remember, enjoying international cuisines as a vegetarian is all about being open-minded, willing to explore new ingredients, and being creative in the kitchen. With the wealth of vegetarian options available globally, you can savor the flavors and delights of different cultures while staying true to your dietary choices.

7.8 How can I stay motivated and sustain my vegetarian lifestyle long term?

Maintaining motivation and sustaining a vegetarian lifestyle is essential, and we will provide practical tips and advice to help you stay on track. From setting realistic goals to seeking support and celebrating your progress, you will learn how to cultivate a positive mindset and embrace the long-term benefits of a vegetarian lifestyle.

Sustaining a vegetarian lifestyle long term requires motivation and a positive mindset. Here are some strategies to help you stay motivated and committed:

1.Revisit your reasons: Remind yourself of why you chose to adopt a vegetarian lifestyle. Whether it's for ethical, environmental, health, or personal reasons, reconnecting with your motivations can reignite your passion and commitment.

2.Educate yourself: Stay informed about the benefits of vegetarianism. Read books, articles, and watch documentaries about vegetarianism, nutrition, and the impact of food choices. The more you learn, the more empowered and motivated you will feel.

3.Connect with the community: Surround yourself with like-minded individuals who share your values and dietary choices. Join vegetarian or vegan groups, attend local meetups or events, and engage in online communities. Sharing experiences, recipes, and challenges with others can provide support, inspiration, and a sense of belonging.

4.Try new recipes and cuisines: Keep your vegetarian meals exciting and diverse by exploring new recipes and cuisines. Experiment with different ingredients, flavors, and cooking techniques. There are countless vegetarian recipes available online, in cookbooks, and through cooking apps. Challenge yourself to try at least one new recipe each week.

5.Plan and prepare meals: Plan your meals in advance and make a grocery list to ensure you have all the necessary ingredients. Having a well-stocked pantry and fridge with vegetarian-friendly options makes it easier to prepare nutritious meals. Meal prepping can also save time and make healthy choices more convenient.

6.Focus on nutrition: Ensure you're getting all the necessary nutrients from your vegetarian diet. Pay attention to sources of protein, iron, calcium, vitamin B12, omega-3 fatty acids, and other key nutrients. Consider consulting with a registered dietitian to create a well-balanced meal plan that meets your nutritional needs.

7.Celebrate milestones and successes: Acknowledge and celebrate the progress you've made as a vegetarian. Whether it's reaching a specific time milestone, trying new foods, or making positive changes in your health, give yourself credit for your achievements. Rewarding yourself along the way can help maintain motivation.

8.Practice self-care: Take care of your overall well-being by practicing self-care. Get enough sleep, engage in regular physical activity, manage stress, and prioritize self-reflection. Taking care of yourself holistically will contribute to your motivation and resilience.

9.Be kind to yourself: Understand that nobody is perfect, and slip-ups or challenges may happen along the way. If you make a mistake or have a moment of weakness, don't beat yourself up. Instead, use it as a learning experience and an opportunity to grow.

10.Stay focused on the bigger picture: Remember the positive impact you're making through your vegetarian lifestyle. Reflect on the ethical, environmental, and personal benefits of your choices. By staying focused on the bigger picture, you can find motivation to sustain your vegetarian lifestyle long term.

Remember, sustaining a vegetarian lifestyle is a journey, and It's okay to have ups and downs. Stay flexible, adapt as needed, and keep your goals and values at the forefront. With commitment, motivation, and a positive mindset, you can embrace and sustain your vegetarian lifestyle for the long term.

Conclusion:

In this chapter, we addressed frequently asked questions about vegetarianism, offering insights and practical guidance. By understanding the nutritional aspects, exploring protein sources, and addressing concerns about iron, calcium, and omega-3s, you can feel confident in your vegetarian diet. Additionally, we discussed considerations for children, pregnant women, and handling social situations as a vegetarian. Armed with this knowledge, you can navigate your vegetarian journey with ease and enjoy the diverse and delicious world of plant-based cuisine. In the concluding chapter, we will reflect

Chapter 8:

Conclusion

As we come to the end of this book, we hope that you have gained valuable insights and practical tips to help you embrace the vegetarian lifestyle. We have explored the benefits of vegetarianism, the science behind it, and how to transition to a plant-based diet.

In the first chapter, we introduced the concept of vegetarianism and its growing popularity. We also discussed the reasons people choose to become vegetarians and the potential health and environmental benefits.

In chapter 2, we explored the different types of vegetarianism, including lacto-ovo, vegan, and flexitarian. We also looked at the history of vegetarianism and its cultural significance.

Chapter 3 focused on getting started with vegetarianism, including practical tips for transitioning, meal planning, and grocery shopping. We also discussed common challenges and how to overcome them.

In chapter 4, we delved into the science of nutrition and meal planning for vegetarians. We highlighted essential nutrients, such as protein, iron, calcium, and omega-3 fatty acids, and how to incorporate them into a vegetarian diet.

Chapter 5 provided delicious vegetarian recipes, from breakfast dishes to main courses and desserts. We also discussed the versatility of vegetarian ingredients and how to adapt international cuisines to suit a plant-based diet.

Chapter 6 addressed overcoming challenges and staying motivated on your vegetarian journey. We provided strategies for dealing with social situations, seeking support, and cultivating a positive mindset.

In chapter 7, we addressed frequently asked questions about vegetarianism, including nutritional concerns, protein sources, handling social situations, and sustainability.

In conclusion, "Living Green: Embracing the Vegetarian Lifestyle" invites readers on a journey towards a more sustainable, compassionate, and healthy way of living. Throughout this book, we have explored the multitude of benefits associated with vegetarianism, from reducing our ecological footprint to improving our overall well-being. By choosing a vegetarian lifestyle, we have the power to make a positive impact on the planet, animals, and ourselves.

We have delved into the foundations of vegetarianism, providing insights into the ethical considerations, nutritional aspects, and practical tips for transitioning to a plant-based diet. By understanding the underlying principles and embracing the diverse range of vegetarian options, readers have gained the tools necessary to embark on their own unique vegetarian journey.

Throughout the pages of this book, we have highlighted the importance of balance, variety, and mindfulness in creating a nutritionally complete vegetarian diet. We have explored the rich tapestry of vegetarian cuisine, showcasing the delicious flavors and culinary possibilities that await. From mouthwatering plant-based recipes to guidance on meal planning, readers have been equipped with the knowledge and inspiration to create delectable, nourishing meals.

But this book goes beyond mere recipes and dietary advice. It has encouraged readers to cultivate a positive mindset, embrace flexibility, and overcome challenges as they navigate their vegetarian lifestyle. From strategies for social situations to dealing with cravings, the guidance provided here has empowered readers to confidently assert their dietary choices while fostering meaningful connections with others.

As we conclude this journey, let us remember that being a vegetarian is not just about what we eat— it is a conscious choice that extends to every aspect of our lives. It is about aligning our values with our actions, being mindful of the impact of our choices, and striving for a more compassionate and sustainable world.

May this book serve as a source of inspiration, information, and guidance, empowering readers to embrace the vegetarian lifestyle wholeheartedly. Let us embark on this journey together, celebrating the joys and triumphs that come with living green, nourishing our bodies, and making a positive difference in the world.

Remember, transitioning to a vegetarian lifestyle is a journey, not a destination. Be patient with yourself, celebrate your progress, and stay motivated. The benefits of vegetarianism are worth the effort, both for your health and the environment.

We hope this book has been a helpful resource on your vegetarian journey. Thank you for joining us, and we wish you all the best on your path towards a healthy, sustainable, and fulfilling plant-based lifestyle.

www.ingramcontent.com/pod-product-compliance
Lightning Source LLC
Chambersburg PA
CBHW072249260726

48657CB00005BA/1714